Book 1:

Essential Oils & Weight Loss for Beginners

BY LINDSEY P

&

Book 2:

Essential Oils & Aromatherapy for Beginners

BY LINDSEY P

Book 1:

Essential Oils & Weight Loss for Beginners

BY LINDSEY P

Ultimate Guide to Losing Weight, Increasing Energy, Balancing Metabolism & Appetite Using Essential Oils & Aromatherapy

Essential Oils
&
Weight Loss
For Beginners

Ultimate Guide to Losing Weight, Increasing
Energy, Balancing Metabolism & Appetite Using
Essential Oils and Aromatherapy

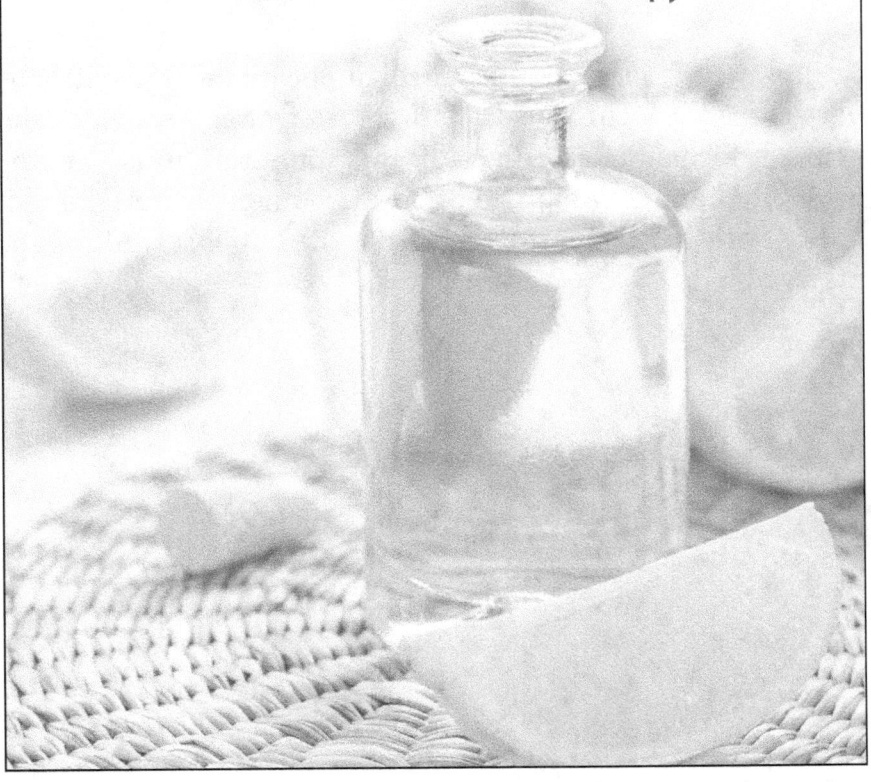

Table Of Contents

Introduction

I want to thank you and congratulate you for downloading the book, "Essential Oils & Weight Loss for Beginners".

This book contains proven steps and strategies on how to make essentials oils work for you to help you conquer the battle against the weighing scale and measuring tape and to increase your energy and balance your metabolism.

It might sound a little far-fetched to hear that certain essential oils can actually help you to fight off your bulges. However, it is indeed possible! By the end of reading this book, you will find yourself more prepared and equipped to make essential oils work to your advantage. Read on to find out how orange peel essential oils can help turn your orange-peel skin into a cellulite-free smooth and toned skin.

Thanks again for downloading this book, I hope you enjoy it!

Chapter 1: Essential Oils Basics

Before you get to learn which essential oils can help you in weight loss and how these can accomplish that, let us discuss first just what exactly essential oils are.

Essential oils are concentrated liquids that have a tendency to not absorb water or to not dissolve in or mix with water, it also has botanical aroma compounds that evaporate readily at normal temperature or pressure.

Oils from different kinds of plants are termed "essential" because it contains the essence or specific scent of the plant from which it was taken. It does not mean that it is essential or a must for one's health, but it sure can help us in more ways than one.

Distillation is the most common way used to extract essential oils from plants. Lavender, peppermint, and eucalyptus essential oils are the most commonly distilled oils. The different parts of the plant where the extract is to be taken from, like the roots, leaves, flowers, and others, are put inside a distillation apparatus, known as an alembic. It is then put over water and then heated. As the water's temperature rises, it will produce steam that will pass through the part of the plant, which will then vaporize the volatile elements in it. Then the vaporized compounds will then flow through a cooling coil, which will make it condense and return to a liquid state. Then the extracted liquid will then be collected in a container.

The less common processes are expression, which involves pressing the plants in a pressing device or machine to squeeze out the oils. Most citrus peels, like orange, lemon, and grapefruit, are expressed to get their essential oils. They can either be pressed mechanically or through cold-press. The peel of citrus fruits yield a large quantity of oil. In addition, growing and harvesting them takes very low cost. For this reason, essential oils from citrus fruits are less expensive compared to the cost of other essential oils.

Another way to get essential oils from plants is solvent extraction, which involves separating compounds using a funnel that separates it into two different liquids depending on their solubility. Most commonly, flowers undergo this process as they do not have enough volatile compounds for expression. Moreover, the chemical elements of flowers are too delicate and are readily denatured when heated at high temperatures using the process of steam distillation. Therefore, extraction through the use of solvents such as supercritical carbon dioxide is used to get the oils from the flowers.

Essential oils, also known as plant extracts, are used in cosmetics, soaps, perfumes, food and beverage flavoring, and other scented products. Although essential oils are not a requirement for the health, these have been applied medically throughout history as hair and skin treatments, cancer cures, aromatherapy, and others.

Western and Oriental medicine practitioners often argue about the efficacy of essential oils. Oriental or alternative medicine claims essential oils as having curative effects and many can testify to having been directly benefited by essential oils. When giving or being given acupressure or different kinds of massages, essential oils are used directly on the skin to be absorbed through the pores or diffused by nebulizers or burned as a candle or incense to be absorbed through the lungs.

If you would like to know how certain essential oils can help you to increase your metabolism, boost your energy, and help you lose weight, then please read on to the next chapter.

Chapter 2: How They Work for You

It is absolutely true that using certain essential oils can help you burn fat. However, nothing quite beats good old-fashioned proper diet and exercise. Discretion should be used when using essential oils to aid in weight loss. Never should one imagine or expect that certain essential oils are enough to keep your body fit and trimmed while you overeat and under-exercise.

That being said though, essential oils coupled with proper diet and exercise can do wonders for your body. Losing weight is not just about what you eat or what you do. It is also about how you feel about your body and about yourself.

Certain essential oils can help you when you are overeating because of certain events or experiences in your life. Let's face it. We eat our feelings every now and then. Whenever we are sorely distressed over something, we will almost instantly head to our favorite comfort food restaurant or food stall to eat a devilishly delicious and decadent chocolate cake or some hot and crispy deep fried poultry and root crops. Whichever the case, essential oils can give you comfort from whatever it is you are going through that makes you overeat with zero calories.

There are no particular essential oils that burn fat directly. However, certain essential oils can boost your metabolism, which in turn can help you in your weight loss goal and in cutting your body's fat deposits. Therefore, you must choose essential oils that aid in boosting your energy and metabolism.

Some of these energy-boosting and metabolism-balancing essential oils include citrus fruits (like oranges, lemons, bergamot, and grapefruits), herbs (like rosemary, sandalwood, and basil), and spices (like ginger, peppermint, and cinnamon).

There are many different ways in which you can mix and use these essential oils to your benefit depending on what you need them for. In the next chapter, we will talk about essential oils from citrus fruits.

Chapter 3: Citrus Essential Oils

It has long been proven by scientists that there is a strong link between what you smell, how you feel, and what eating pattern you have. Often, we take our senses for granted and do not realize just how strongly it affects our brain and behavior. You would agree that there is more than one time when your stomach grumbles like it is hungry when in fact, you just ate a short while ago and you are not actually hungry. Steadily inhaling citrus scents can help deceive our brain into thinking that our stomachs are full and therefore stopping it from sending signals to the brain that it is hungry.

The citrus family is a huge family. Citrus fruits have always benefited mankind in more ways than one. In this chapter, we will highlight the weight loss benefits of using essential oils from citrus fruits.

ORANGE. First on our list is the humble yet mighty and versatile orange. Different types of orange peels can yield their essential oils through the process of cold expression. Essential oils from different kinds of oranges are the most commonly added ingredients to various beauty products. Anti-aging creams, energizing body lotions, refreshing body wash variants, and other body care products use orange essential oils. Likewise, household items such as scented candles, aerosol deodorizing sprays for the rooms, and other scented products use orange essential oils.

Orange essential oils are also quite often used in pastries and other types of dishes as a flavoring and you would have ingested it more often than you are aware of. That being said though, you might become skeptical as to the efficacy of it since you have not felt directly any of its supposed properties in aiding you to lose weight and control your appetite.

The main reason for this is that the amount you absorb or consume is not enough for you to be able to feel the supposed effects. It can only act as a mood booster but that is pretty much the best you can get out of it. In order for you to feel the weight loss benefits, the orange essential oil must be in pure organic and undiluted form. That is why it is important to buy the pure, undiluted oils from trusted organic sources.

However, you must not confuse the fruit with the oil. The orange fruit is absolutely delicious and refreshing to the taste buds to eat. But the pure, undiluted orange oil is not to be eaten the way you would the fruit. To be able to benefit from the oil, you must use it in an aromatherapy session to help you control your cravings and cope with the everyday stress you encounter that might lead you to overeat.

You can put the orange essential oil in a diffuser to give a lingering, pleasant scent that everyone in the room can savor while the scent fills the room. If you are out and about, you can also bring a portable diffuser or inhaler so you can steadily inhale the refreshing scent of oranges for about five minutes to curb your cravings anytime you get them.

GRAPEFRUIT. The next one in line in the citrus family is the grapefruit. Grapefruit essential oils can stop your body from retaining water, which is one of the main causes of bloating, and can also dissolve fat in the body. The essential oil accomplishes this by releasing the stored fat into the bloodstream so your body can dissolve and absorb it and turn it into energy, helping you to feel energized. So you can say goodbye to your cellulites and say hello to toned thighs and arms.

Like orange essential oils, grapefruit essential oils can also be a strong suppressant for your cravings. It can help you feel fuller for longer. You can put a few drops of the grapefruit essential oil into your diffuser or inhaler to stop any hunger pangs from making you reach for another bag of chips. Another way is to put a drop of the essential oil in 8 ounces of drinking water to drink before you have your lunch or dinner. This will stop you from eating more than you should.

Grapefruit essential oils also help uplift your thoughts and moods. Improved moods can help you deal with stress better and help you have a better acceptance of yourself and your body, which can save you from developing any eating disorders, be it eating too much or too little.

You can mix different essentials oils as well to achieve better results. When you encounter extra stressful days that make you want to dive into a tub of vanilla ice cream, why not dive into your bath tub instead? Try mixing about eight drops of grapefruit essential oil and five drops of ginger essential oil to about two ounces of olive or sweet almond oil into your bath water and soak away to refreshment and relaxation.

The different essential oils you can mix together to relieve stress are lemon, chamomile, lavender, grapefruit, and jasmine essential oils. These essential oils have a calming effect. If you are depressed, uplifting and mood-boosting mixes can be of rose, sandalwood, orange, lavender, grapefruit, and jasmine essential oils. If you are feeling anxious, you can arrange for a massage and add a mixture or bergamot, sandalwood, rose, and lavender to your massage oil or as an incense to chase your anxieties away.

LEMON. Lemon essential oil is extracted from lemon rinds using cold press. It gently detoxifies the body. It relieves the body of some intestinal parasites that contribute to ill digestive health. Lemon has the ability to cleanse the body from toxins because of the antioxidant limonene. You can add a drop of lemon essential oil in a glass of water for a refreshing and uplifting drink. As with the abovementioned citrus fruits, lemon essential oil shares the same benefits for people wanting to lose weight and control their eating habits.

BERGAMOT. Bergamot is about the size of a typical orange but with a yellow rind like a lemon's. It is also used in many medicinal concoctions. Bergamot essential oils are strongly sedative and is therefore calming and best to use when you are stressed or tense that you want to reach for something decadent. So instead of letting sweets and simple sugars calm your nerves, let bergamot essential oils work for you. You will get the same calming effect without any added calories to your diet.

When paired with lavender essential oils, the calming or sedative effect will be more powerful. You can take a clean cloth and put a few drops of bergamot on it then steadily inhale it to help you relax when you are stressed out or when you get the urge to eat when you know you shouldn't. You can also dilute a drop of the oil in a teaspoon of honey and take it as you would cough syrup. Or you can make a calming yet delicious drink by diluting a drop of the oil in a small glass of almond or soy milk.

Well, now that you are acquainted with the citrus family, let us now get to know the other essential oils that will become your best friends in your war against cellulites.

Chapter 4: Non-citrus Essential Oils

In this chapter, we are going to talk about the not-so-citrus essential oils and how they can help us in expelling adipose tissues that are overstaying in our bodies.

PEPPERMINT. There is a part of your brain that tells you that your stomach is now filled with your mother's special meatloaf and that it can't accommodate anymore meatloaf. But sometimes, or should I say most of the time, we ignore what our brain tells us and listen to our eyes and taste buds telling us to eat more. Peppermint specifically works on that part of your brain to make it keep telling you that you are indeed full.

In addition, your tummy will love peppermint because it has proven itself as a great helper for digestion. It resolves a wide variety of digestive ailments. It can help you out if you are having problems with candida, as it is often a big influence in your losing or gaining weight. Moreover, when you are under heavy emotions like depression or anxiety, it can uplift and lighten your mood and motivate you to be more optimistic. And most importantly, peppermint tastes amazing and will let you give a minty fresh kiss to your special someone as well.

Before you eat anything, put a couple of drops of peppermint essential oil to a clean cloth or a cotton pad and steadily breathe in vapors. You can also put the drops in a diffuser and inhale your way to a reduced appetite. Likewise, you can put a drop of the peppermint oil in a glass of water for a refreshing drink before each meal. You can also pair it with lemon to get the most energizing and waistline-reducing effect.

SANDALWOOD. Sandalwood essential oils also have calming sedative properties that can help you control your eating habits when you are undergoing stressful situations. Sandalwood helps you combat negative feelings and actions. The feeling of having conquered negativity with relieve you of the stress you were having and so relieving you as well of the impulse to eat something comforting like you beloved mother's macaroni and cheese.

Sandalwood essential oils may be used with a diffuser and constantly inhaling the vapors. You can also dilute a drop of the sandalwood oil in a drop of extra virgin olive oil and then apply it directly on your feet or stomach for faster absorption. You can also take it like you would any medical syrup by adding a drop of sandalwood essential oil to a teaspoon of honey. You can also make a delicious drink by mixing a drop of the sandalwood oil to a small glass of rice milk.

GINGER. The lowly ginger is quite famous in Asian cuisine for being tummy-friendly. It is this spicy yet mildly sweet ingredient that makes Asian dishes taste really good. But its being tummy-friendly is not just because it makes dishes taste awesome. It is also loved by your stomach because of its anti-inflammatory and anti-bacterial properties that makes the stomach healthy and in tip-top shape.

In addition, ginger also has a warming effect on the body because of its being mildly spicy, stimulating the body, especially the nervous system. Ginger essential oil has been dubbed as the "oil of empowerment" as it gives off a mild heat that stimulates our inner strength, energizing and empowering the body and the mind.

To get the full benefit of ginger essential oil, you can put a couple of drops in a diffuser and inhale the vapors as you would any other essential oils that we have already discussed. You can also apply it directly to your skin or by diluting it first in coconut oil if you have sensitive skin. You can do a skin test first by applying it to your forearm to see if you are sensitive to it or not.

CINNAMON. Cinnamon is known to increase the weight loss effectiveness of all the other essential oils you have read about in this book. Diabetics can find comfort in knowing that cinnamon has been discovered to trigger healthy levels of insulin in the body. It also improves digestion and blood circulation. Its antioxidant properties help in gently detoxifying the body and stimulating the immune system to get to fight against invaders that try to give us colds and flu.

Cinnamon essential oil taken from the cinnamon leaves and twigs through steam distillation has a mildly spicy and musky scent. Cinnamon is great in aromatherapy. However, cinnamon oil from the cinnamon bark in not usually used in aromatherapy. Much like ginger essential oils, cinnamon essential oils are also mildly spicy and so it warms up the body as well and fights against exhaustion and depression by empowering the body.

In aromatherapy, you can put a few drops of the cinnamon essential oil in burners or vaporizers to be inhaled steadily to calm you and take your mind off eating out of stress. You can also dilute the oil in your bath water as you soak all your worries away. In addition, you can also simultaneously fight off any outwardly infections while soaking in your cinnamon infused bath water because of the cinnamon oil's antiseptic properties.

Chapter 5: A Helper and Complement

These essential oils that we have discussed in this book will only be effective if you work hard at your goal as well. Remember that nothing can replace proper diet and regular exercise to help you keep fit and healthy. But these essential oils can greatly help you in your struggle against whether to pick up that mouth-watering sandwich and take a bite off of it when you are not genuinely hungry.

These previously mentioned essential oils will boost you the two other main weapons in your war against excess fat. These essential oils have different properties that work to help you in breaking down fat in order to be fully absorbed by your body and turned into energy. They help curb your appetite and your "midnight-snack" cravings. They affect the part of the brain to help you relax and calm down instead of converting your anxieties and stresses into overeating.

Of course, disciplining yourself to eat the right kinds of food and to have a regular exercise program is difficult at first. You might be dreading or avoiding having to eat healthy food or having to go to the gym or just increase your daily physical activity. It might be the very reason that you have bought this book trying to find a way to lose weight without having to follow a proper diet and a regular exercise plan.

Well, following the instructions above and using essential oils alone in your goal of losing weight is indeed a possibility. It is not impossible. However, it is not enough and all the more so if you continue to live a sedentary lifestyle and choose unhealthy kinds of food. There should be balance in everything. One way or another, you are going to have to face the consequences of your actions (or for that matter, lack of action).

It is not at all daunting to follow a proper diet plan and a regular exercise program. But first, you have to want to make yourself healthier. Without your will and motivation, you most probably will not succeed. Moreover, you need to be consistent and steady with your routine to reach your goal of losing weight and keeping fit. If you are not consistent, you will undergo a yo-yo pattern, in which you will lose weight when you are motivated and gain weight when you are not.

It is not only bad for your health, it is also bad for your physical appearance as well because a yo-yo diet will ruin the elasticity of your skin causing it to have stretch marks and that will not be a very nice sight to see. Losing weight gradually coupled with good exercise will give your skin time to adjust to fit your new size, reducing the possibility of stretch marks and skin flaps that are commonly seen in people undergoing crash diets.

The food you eat also plays a big role in your goal to losing weight. Aside from keeping your body healthy in general, vitamins in fruits and vegetables, particularly vitamins A and E, will greatly increase your skins elasticity and give you a rosy glow on your cheeks suggesting you are indeed in the "pink of health".

The essential oils discussed in this book will be your ally in keeping a regular exercise routine. Orange and peppermint essential oils will perk you up and keep you feeling energized and motivated to follow your exercise program. Cinnamon and ginger essential oils will empower you to keep going even when you feel like you can't go on anymore.

Sandalwood and bergamot essential oils will calm and relax your nerves when you are feeling stressed out so you can win against the temptations of rich desserts and deep fried foods. And the best part about these essential oils is that it gives no side effects as it is pure and having no caffeine, no sugar, no preservatives.

A word of caution though. You may find some shops selling essential oils, usually containing a mixture of grapefruit, coconut, cedar, and other essential oils, claiming to burn fat. It would be great for calming and energizing you as discussed above. However, these cannot really help you to break down fat or cellulite in your body. It may temporarily make your skin look firmer because it hydrates your skin, but it is not a permanent fix.

It is better to research and experiment about which aromatherapy works best for you. Make sure that you do your homework and that you know how to properly use diffusers or inhalers to get the best out of your essential oils. When applying the essential oils directly on your body, make sure you dilute it first in a carrier oil such as virgin olive oil or coconut oil. Remember as well that some essential oils can be toxic to you if you directly ingest it. Always keep them in a safe place away from young children. Unless you have been using the essential oils for some time, only follow specific recipes to make sure it is safe for you.

Chapter 6: A Look in the Mirror

A mirror helps you to see yourself to check if you need to adjust your tie, if you need to reapply your lipstick, or if you have a piece of red bell pepper stuck to your teeth. But sometimes people forget to look at their inner mirror to check if the way they think or see things is correct. You need to take a good long look at yourself as well.

You need to honestly ask yourself whether you are doing this for yourself, to make yourself a better and healthier person or whether you are doing this just to please someone else. It is true that you need to present yourself well and make sure you look presentable when dealing with other people. But you should not change yourself just to please someone who does not genuinely care about you.

The motivation to lose weight should come from you, not from somebody else. Moreover, you should do it for the right reasons. When you are guided by a proper motivation and you have the right reasons to embark on the journey to weight loss, you will have more stability and consistency all throughout.

You will have a reason to go on even when you encounter setbacks in your goals, such as an unexpected dinner celebration for your friend's promotion or a relapse into pigging out during a family reunion, which ruins your carefully planned out diet, or a surprise added workload, which meant you would have to give up going to the gym for a few days to accommodate the added workload.

You need to be able to motivate yourself to continue even when setbacks happen. However, you will not always be strong. Therefore, having a loved one or a friend know of your goals and asking for their support will greatly help you win the war against your bulges. You can also have a "weight loss buddy" whom you can be with as you journey towards a better health and a better self.

Having someone to exercise and eat proper amounts and right kinds of food with will make exercising and dieting less boring and tiresome. Knowing that you are in this together will empower you more while you let the essential oils work their magic to boost your energy. You can take essential oil-infused baths together or have your massages using your favorite essential oils together.

Not only will you be benefited by your regular exercise program, your proper healthy diet, and the essential oils we have discussed in this book, but you will also be benefited by the soothing and calming effect of human connection. All these things add up to make your whole weight loss journey more pleasant. Remember that those are puzzle pieces that need to be put together in order for you to complete the picture.

Conclusion

Thank you again for downloading this book!

I hope this book was able to help you to realize the hidden potential of certain essential oils in weight loss, in increasing your body's energy, in uplifting your mood and countenance, and in improving your overall well-being.

The next step is to apply what you have learned in this book and to get you going on your way to physical fitness and better health. Remember that these facts about the essential oils mentioned above will be useless if you do not work hard and work steady. Avoid the yo-yo and crash diets. Slow and steady wins the race too. And in the race to weight loss, the fast and furious method won't really cut it. Take your time and enjoy your journey to a thinner and more healthy you!

Finally, if you enjoyed this book, please take the time to share your thoughts and post a review on Amazon. We do our best to reach out to readers and provide the best value we can. Your positive review will help us achieve that. It'd be greatly appreciated!

Thank you and good luck!

Book 2:

Essential Oils & Aromatherapy for Beginners

BY LINDSEY P

Secrets to Beauty, Health and Weight Loss Using Proven Essential Oil and Aromatherapy Recipes

2nd Edition

Essential Oils
&
Aromatherapy
For Beginners

Secrets To Beauty, Health And Weight Loss Using
Proven Essential Oil And Aromatherapy Recipes

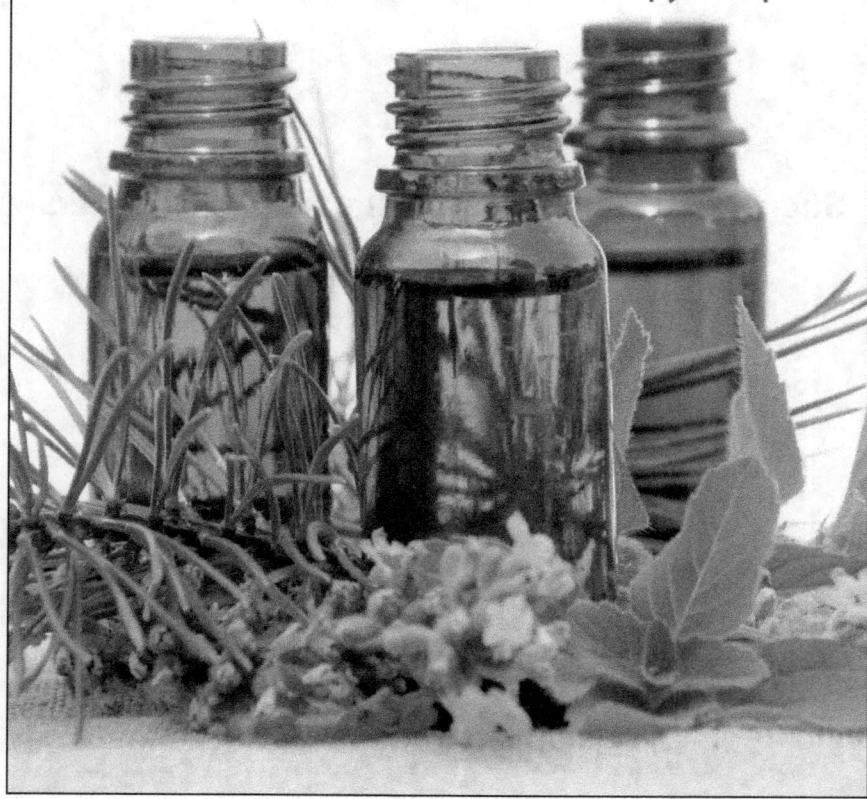

Table Of Contents

Introduction

I want to thank you and congratulate you for downloading the book, *"Essential Oils & Aromatherapy for Beginners: Secrets to Beauty, Health and Weight Loss Using Proven Essential Oil and Aromatherapy Recipes "*.

This book contains proven steps and strategies on how to use essential oils, either pure or in combination, to solve common problems in beauty and health. Using essential oils as opposed to commercial formulations for your various problems can help you maintain an all-natural lifestyle. This is good for the environment, for yourself and, in certain circumstances, for your wallet too.

Thanks again for downloading this book, I hope you enjoy it!

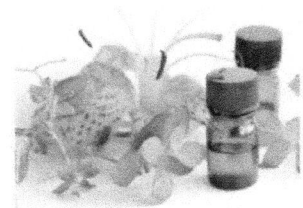

Chapter 1 – Using Essential Oils

Essential oils have been used for centuries in many cultures to cure common health ailments, solve various household problems, soothe the soul, make someone fall in love with you, drive evil spirits away and many others. While some of these uses may have been proven false by science, many are retained particularly for beauty and over-all health.

Technically speaking, an essential oil is the oily liquid that is distilled from the whole plant or certain parts of it. The color, oiliness and viscosity of an essential oil vary depending on the plant. Some essential oils feel like water and are as clear as water while some will feel oily and will have a yellowish or brownish color.

Essential oils are given that name because they are, in a sense, the essence of the plant. Think of them as the concentrated goodness of the plant. This is why they ought to be used sparingly and also why they can, especially for topical uses, be good for your wallet. Depending on the brand and on the essential oil, a 30 ml. bottle will usually cost around US $20, but since you only use 1 to 2 drops at a time, that small bottle will go a long way.

Essential oils will have their own scent and are commonly used in making fragrance, but they should be differentiated from fragrance oils which are artificially scented oils. The latter are commonly used in oil burners, for potpourri and sometimes for cheap scented soaps and candles. To the uninitiated, fragrance oils and products made with them can seem like a better buy because they are cheaper, but there will be a difference in the scent of true essential oil and artificial fragrance oil. The longer you have used true essential oils, the more you can distinguish between them and artificial scents.

Some proponents of aromatherapy will insist that only true essential oils will give actual benefits. This is debatable since there have been no serious studies made on this yet. If you are using fragrance oils for your oil burner or for making candles because they are cheaper, and you think the scent is giving you some benefits, then by all means continue to use this fragrance oil. However, I will encourage you to splurge on true essential oil to learn the difference. Soon, you might find that true essential oil gives you better benefits and you will find that the difference in cost is worth it.

Fragrance oils can be used safely for oil burners and scenting potpourri, BUT they should never be used topically on the skin. Some cheap kinds of soaps which are scented with fragrance oils may not irritate the skin since only a small amount is used, but if you use pure fragrance oils directly on 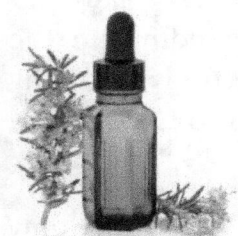 the skin, even the most insensitive skins can experience irritation. Also, since fragrance oils are only artificially scented oils, you will not get any skin care benefits from them as you would from true essential oils.

If cost is really a problem with essential oils, you should know that they are concentrated and are usually used diluted with vegetable oil. This is commonly called 'carrier oil' because they 'carry' the essential oil. The best carrier oils are those which do not have a natural scent like jojoba or grape seed oil. These oils also feel light on the skin since they have a similar composition to sebum or our skin's natural oil. For drier skins, olive, rose hip, coconut or avocado oil may be better options but they can have a natural scent of their own and can affect the overall scent of your essential oil. We will further discuss carrier oils per se in chapter 4.

You need to experiment on the right ratio of essential oil and carrier oil for your specific skin type. Always start with a 1:1 ratio then add more carrier oil if you experience irritation or add more essential oil if you are not seeing the results you want.

Always keep your essential oils in a cool dark place regardless whether they are diluted or pure. Take note that most essential oils are stored in dark bottles. As much as possible, when making your own combinations, use dark bottles as well. Also, it is better to buy small amounts of essential oil and wait until this is used up before buying a new one. This way you can be assured that the essential oil you use is always fresh.

The potency of essential oils must always be stressed since you might hurt yourself if you are not careful. Certain essential oils can also be extremely irritating to the eyes and mouth when they are used near these areas. Those with sensitive skins must be particularly careful because they can still experience irritation even when essential oils are used diluted.

Also, it is possible to be allergic to essential oils. If you have a lot of allergies, it is better to do a skin test first before using the essential oil for your topical skin care. If you will not use the essential oil for topical purposes, then you need not do a skin test.

To do a skin test, apply a small drop of the pure essential oil on a hidden part of the body like the inside of your elbow. Wait for 24 hours to see if any redness or irritation will happen. If you do not experience irritation, you can safely use the essential oil for skin and health care. You should do this for every essential oil you need to use.

There are some who say that even if you experience irritation with the pure oil, you can still use it diluted. If you wish to test this on yourself, do the same skin test described above but dilute the small drop of pure essential oil with the same amount of your choice of carrier oil. However, do not risk doing this if you have extremely sensitive skin.

The succeeding chapters will teach you which essential oils are the best for many problems. It might seem as if you need to buy several bottles of various kinds, but if you read carefully, you will notice that one essential oil can have various uses. For example, lavender essential oil can be used for acne, for calming the mind, for wrinkles and for minor skin burns. Thus, if you are already using this for your acne, you can use the same bottle for other purposes as well.

This can be another reason why it is better to buy true essential oil instead of fragrance oils even if you initially had no intention of using the fragrance oil topically. If you bought a cheap bottle of lavender fragrance oil, you can only use this for scenting your room, and it will be an inferior scent at that. If you buy true lavender essential oil, the whole family can use that single bottle *and* you get a better scent.

Chapter 2 – Skin Care

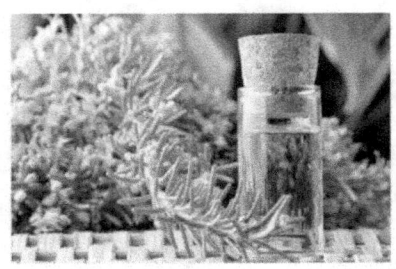

There are various skin care problems which essential oils can cure. The most common are acne, wrinkles or aging skin, fungal infections, psoriasis and eczema, and minor skin burns and wounds. We will discuss each problem in turn.

For acne, the most effective essential oils are tea tree oil, lavender and neem oil. These essential oils effectively kill acne bacteria. Depending on the severity of your acne and the sensitivity of your skin, use the pure essential oil or appropriately diluted. The lighter vegetable oils like jojoba and grape seed are the better choice for oily skins, but if you have normal or dry skin and just happen to suffer from acne, coconut oil can be a good choice since it can add anti-bacterial properties to your essential oil solution.

What you choose will depend on how fast you wish your acne to be gone and your scent preference. Tea tree oil is generally considered the fastest acting essential oil for acne followed by lavender oil and neem oil. However, take note that even tea tree oil will act slower compared to commercial acne treatments containing benzoyl peroxide and salicylic acid. If so, what can be a reason for you to choose essential oils? As mentioned in the introduction, you can opt to choose essential oils because you prefer a natural lifestyle. Also, in the long run, essential oils can be cheaper because you use only a very small amount.

Regarding scent, tea tree oil is spicy and woody, lavender is soothing and feminine while neem oil is the worst smelling. The scent of neem oil has been compared to a skunk and to stale urine, but it has an added benefit of smoothing out fine lines and wrinkles. Thus, if you have mature skin and suffer from acne, neem oil can be the better option. The scent can be minimized by your carrier oil and by a small amount of either lavender or tea tree oil.

For wrinkles or aging skin, the best essential oils are the following: clary sage, frankincense, geranium, lavender, lemon, patchouli, rose, rosemary, sandalwood and ylang-ylang. Like with acne, choose your essential oil depending on your preferred scent, and if you have sensitive skin, depending on what does not give you irritation. You can also combine these oils to create a unique scent. Rose and patchouli will give you a sophisticated feminine scent while lavender and lemon will give a fresh and stimulating albeit still feminine scent.

You can apply these essential oils with your choice of carrier oil as described for acne. Since aging skin is usually dry, it is better to use olive, avocado or coconut oil. Argan and rosehip oils are more expensive options but they have additional anti-aging properties.

If you prefer a cream texture for your anti-aging skin care, you can also add shea butter or cocoa butter to your carrier oil. Use ¼ cup of shea or cocoa butter with ¼ cup of your choice of carrier oil, then add 10 to 20 drops of your choice of essential oil or a combination. Melt this over a low fire, stir well then pour into a sterilized glass jar. Allow to cool before putting the lid on. Keep this jar in a cool, dark place. If you live in a hot climate or if it is currently the summer months, keep this jar in the refrigerator.

Alternatively, coconut oil by itself can become solid depending on the temperature. You can whip ½ cup of solid coconut oil before adding 10 to 20 drops of essential oil. Stir well. Keep this in a clean jar in the refrigerator so it will not liquefy.

Acne and wrinkles can also benefit from a toner and steam facial using the same essential oils recommended for each problem. To make toner, use distilled water and a sterilized bottle. For every cup of water, add 10 to 15 drops of essential oil. You can also replace the water with strongly brewed tea to add some antioxidant benefits. For acne and for oily skins, you can use commercially available witch hazel solution. Dry skins can use rose water.

A toner can be used to provide extra cleansing or to refresh the face in the middle of the day. If you wish to do the latter, store your toner in a spray bottle. Allow the toner to dry on your face.

To make a steam facial, heat about 5 cups of water then place in a large bowl. Add 5 drops of essential oil then bend over the bowl with a towel over your face. Inhale deeply to obtain the most benefits. For acne, the steam will open your pores and clean the gunk out of them. For wrinkles, the steam will soften your skin and allow it to absorb your moisturizer better. Do this steam facial at least twice a week.

For fungal infections, tea tree oil and neem oil are the best choices. Use them pure to cure your ailment fast or dilute them with a very small amount of carrier oil if you find the scent too strong. You can also apply the essential oil on a cotton pad and use a bandage to keep it in place. To make the scent more appealing, add peppermint oil which can also help alleviate the itch. Also, use coconut oil as your carrier oil since it contains anti-fungal properties.

If your fungal infection is on the foot or hand, you can make a warm soak with essential oils. Pour hot (but not boiling) water onto a basin and add 10 to 20 drops of your chosen essential oil. Carefully lower your hand or foot onto the basin (make sure the water is not boiling hot or else you might burn yourself). Let it sit there until the water cools. Make sure that the infected area is fully submerged. If possible, do this every day before applying more essential oil to the area.

Psoriasis and eczema can be 'cured' the same way as fungal infections. I say 'cured' because these skin ailments are actually auto-immune diseases. They come and go depending on what happens to the whole body. Thus, essential oil 'cures' only alleviate the symptoms like dryness and itch. They can also help prevent infections when the skin is broken after inadvertently scratching too much.

In addition to tea tree oil and neem oil, psoriasis and eczema can be 'cured' with patchouli and peppermint oil.

For minor skin burns and wounds, essential oils can also help to make them heal faster. Take note that we are only talking about *minor* burns and wounds like sun burn and small cuts and grazes. More serious cases should be treated by medical professionals.

The best essential oils for burns are chamomile, lavender, marjoram, peppermint and tea tree oil. Combine 10 to 20 drops with ½ cup of pure aloe vera gel which has been proven to help promote healing or use them with your choice of carrier oil.

Before any treatment, ensure that the area is clean and free from any topical skin formulas like lotions which may interfere with your treatment. Apply your essential oil as often as possible.

For wounds, tea tree, oregano, and thyme oils are good for disinfecting. Apply the essential oil directly on the wound. For already infected wounds, you can use tea tree or lavender oil. After the wound has healed, you can use rose essential oil to help prevent scarring or to make the scar disappear faster.

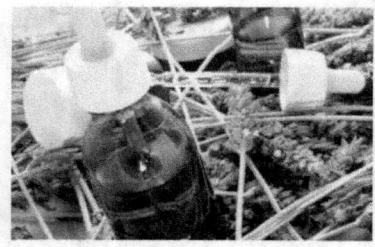

Chapter 3 – Hair Care

Essential oils can also be used to promote great hair. You can encourage faster hair growth, prevent hair damage and prevent frizz. There are also essential oils which can kill head lice and remove scalp psoriasis and dandruff.

For hair growth, rosemary or lavender essential oils are considered the best. Geranium, thyme, sage and ylang-ylang are also good choices. Combine them with your favorite commercial shampoo or apply them directly to the scalp with your favorite carrier oil. The latter will give you better results since you do not rinse off the essential oil. Also, your carrier oil will moisturize your hair and help to prevent frizz. Massage the essential oil with carrier oil onto your scalp for 10 minutes after shampooing. Leave this in your hair for the rest of the day like a conditioning hair oil, or you can do this at night if you dislike putting products on your hair.

For dry hair, use lavender, rosemary or geranium essential oils and combine them with the more emollient carrier oils like olive, coconut, avocado or argan oil. For a deep conditioning treatment, heat this combination until slightly warm then saturate the hair and scalp. Wrap the hair with towels wrung from hot water and leave it for at least an hour. You need to shampoo twice to get all the excess oils out. Do this at least once a month or once a week for best results. Use this same combination daily as a hair oil to prevent frizz.

For head lice, you can choose any of these essential oils: eucalyptus, lemon, thyme, rosemary, tea tree or geranium. Use 1:1 ratio of essential oil with your choice of carrier oil and apply all over the hair and scalp. Leave this for at least half an hour then shampoo it out. Do this until all the lice have died. The length of your treatment will depend on the population of lice on your head.

For scalp psoriasis, use the same recommendations for skin psoriasis but use a lighter carrier oil if you have oily hair.

Lastly, for dandruff, the best essential oils are tea tree oil and eucalyptus. You can use the same method described above for hair growth, but for your carrier oil use coconut oil. This oil has anti-fungal properties which will help kill the fungus which causes dandruff.

Chapter 4 – Carrier Oils

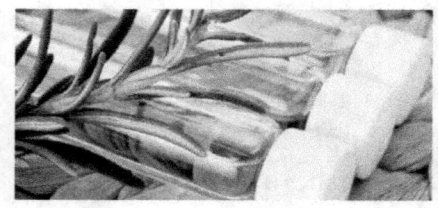

In this chapter, we will discuss carrier oils per se or which carrier oil is best for each specific ailment. If you can pair the best carrier oil with the best essential oil for your problems, then you will be able to solve your problem faster. Carrier oils can be categorized either according to the skin or hair type they are fit for or according to the added advantages they can give like anti-fungal or anti-bacterial properties. Let us start with the first way of categorizing oils.

When we speak of skin or hair type, we talk of dry, normal or oily types. Dry skin is characterized by a lack of sebum or the oil which our skin naturally produces. This sebum is necessary to moisturize the skin and protect it from the elements like too much sun, wind and cold. Those with dry skin find that they easily form fine lines and wrinkles while those with oily skin often look younger during their middle age assuming they do not abuse their bodies with unhealthy habits. Granted that sebum alone is not enough to protect the skin from prolonged exposure to the elements, it at least provides *some* protection. Consider how those with dry skin easily burn from too much sun exposure or easily get itchy after being out too long during a windy or cold day. Dry skin is characterized by tightness and itchiness especially after washing the face with a non-moisturizing cleanser or during cold weather. It can even have tiny, dry flakes of skin hanging on the surface. This skin type is seldom plagued by pimples.

On the other hand, oily skin produces too much sebum. It can look shiny by the middle of the day or even earlier during hot weather when the oil glands are more active. While those with oily skin can look younger even during their older years because their skin is always moisturized, they can be plagued by pimples during their younger years.

Normal skin is considered balanced skin or what the skin should be. It is the ideal skin type and usually does not experience any problems except those which are caused by unhealthy habits like smoking, too much exposure to environmental pollution and an unhealthy diet. If normal skin is well taken care of, it will remain young-looking even until after middle-age.

Unfortunately for us, normal skin is very rare. It is more common for people to have combination skin which means that some areas like the forehead, nose and chin are oilier while the cheek areas are drier.

To check which skin type you have, you need to do this experiment: Wash your face with 10 splashes of water. You need to use water because your choice of cleanser might affect your results. A moisturizing cleanser will add moisture while a cleanser for oily skin might unnecessarily strip your skin. Dry your face with a towel but do not use anything, even toner. If your skin becomes oily all over, i.e. in all parts of your face, after 3 hours or less, you have very oily skin. If your skin becomes oily all over after 6 hours, you have oily skin. If it becomes oily after 8 hours, you have normal skin. If it becomes oily after more than 8 hours, you have normal to dry skin, i.e. dry skin that leans towards being normal. If it does not become oily at all, you have dry skin. If different parts of your face become oily at different times, then use the same criterion described above for those particular parts. Hence it is possible to have a very oily forehead but dry cheeks, and so on.

Take note that I have included the skin types 'very oily' and 'normal to dry.' This is because skin typing is actually better described like a spectrum. Some people will have an oily face after 4 or 5 hours, and some may even become shiny after only 2 hours. Also, your skin type can be affected by the climate you live in. Hot temperatures make the oil glands more active which is why those with normal skin can become oily during summer and dry during winter.

Also, skin type can change depending on your lifestyle choices and age. The skin becomes 10% drier every decade 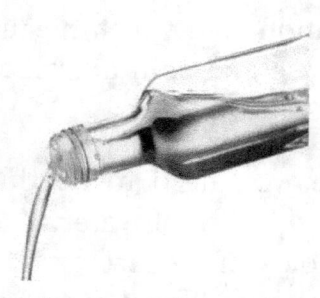 after the age of 20, so a teenager with very oily skin can expect some relief with age. It has also been proven that consuming too much processed foods and animal meats can make the skin oilier while smoking and too much alcohol can make the skin drier. Certain medications can also affect the skin type. In fact, birth control pills have been used by women to control their oil glands in order to keep their acne under control. Topical medications can also be used to control sebum production to help with acne problems.

Meanwhile, when we speak of dry, normal or oily hair, we are actually not speaking of the hair but of the scalp. Hair is also moisturized and protected by sebum which is produced by the scalp. Sebum travels down the hair shaft either naturally or aided by frequent brushing. Dry hair is frizzy and easily tangled because the scalp produces little sebum while oily hair is lank and greasy because there is too much sebum. Normal hair will have a scalp that produces just enough sebum. As with skin, the hair can have very oily and normal to dry types too. The only difference is we do not have combination hair which will mean that some parts of the scalp are oilier than others. While it is possible to have this kind of scalp, it is difficult to check since the oils produced by some parts of the scalp easily spreads to other parts given that the hair strands are very close to each other. Also, as with the skin, the hair type can change with lifestyle and age. Since the scalp is also skin, it will be affected by one's diet and habits. Also, the scalp becomes drier with age which is why old people tend to have brittle hair.

To check which hair type you have, do the same experiment described above for the face, but instead of washing the hair with just water, wash it with a non-conditioning shampoo or a basic shampoo which adds no moisturizers, shine enhancing ingredients or anything else. A good example of this is basic, baby shampoo or mild soap. Rinse the hair well and do not add any hair products. If your hair roots become oily by the end of the day, you have oily hair. If they become oily after 2 days of not washing, you have normal hair. If they never become oily even if you have not washed it for 3 days, you have dry hair.

You need to wait a day or more to check which hair type you have because you cannot easily check your scalp unlike your hair. Also, the sebum produced by your scalp is immediately absorbed by your hair so it will not be easy to know how much sebum it produces.

It is a mistake to think that you will have the same skin and hair type. If it is possible to have combination skin, it is also possible to have a different type for the scalp. Thus, you can have dry hair and oily skin, and vice versa. If so, you might need to use different carrier oils for your face and hair.

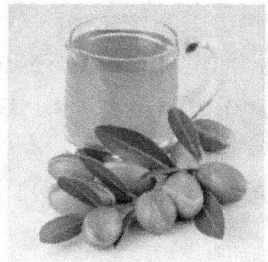

If you have dry skin, the best carrier oils are those which are considered the most emollient. We have mentioned olive, rose hip, coconut and avocado oil in the previous chapters. Argan oil is also a very moisturizing albeit expensive option.

We have mentioned the use of cocoa butter and shea butter instead of carrier oils for a creamier texture. These are carrier substances but they also act like carrier oils in which they 'carry' and dilute the essential oil. Cocoa and shea butter are great options for dry skin, but shea is generally considered more emollient.

When buying butters, you have to make sure that they are not rancid. The best way to do this is to buy from reputable sources which label the date when these butters were made. Also, it is best to buy only the smallest amount possible and to keep it in the refrigerator. You should never use rancid butters especially if you have sensitive skin. Besides the possibility of irritation, they smell bad too. If your butter smells sour or unpleasant, throw it out. Fresh cocoa butter should smell like chocolate while shea should smell sweet and a little bit nutty.

You can also use coconut oil as a 'butter.' In cold temperatures, coconut oil solidifies which make it look like a butter. You can whip this to make it soft then keep your 'butter' in the refrigerator to prevent it from becoming liquid. If you live in colder climates or if summer has passed, your coconut oil 'butter' will likely remain solid even if it is not kept in the refrigerator.

For normal skin, you can use sweet almond, apricot kernel, jojoba or castor oil. The first two will give you a pleasant scent, while the last two will not have much of a scent. Jojoba is considered to be the closest in composition to sebum while castor oil has regenerative, anti-bacterial and anti-fungal properties. We will discuss more on this later.

If you prefer a cream consistency, instead of cocoa or shea butter, you can use beeswax. Though technically beeswax is not a butter but a wax, when mixed with an equal amount of one of the carrier oils listed above, the result is similar to a butter consistency but it is less emollient. This combination is perfect for normal skins.

Using beeswax is slightly more complicated than butters because you always have to melt the wax or else you will not be able to mix it with the other ingredients. Do not use pure beeswax with your essential oils or you will end up with a candle once the wax hardens.

For oily skin, the only carrier oil you must use is grape seed oil. This is the lightest of all the carrier oils. It also has an astringent effect, i.e. it can make the skin drier. As impossible as that sounds considering that we are talking about an oil, those with dry skins who have used grape seed oil report that they ended up with drier skins than they started with. This is because grape seed oil penetrates deeply into the skin and influences the oil glands to produce less sebum. It acts more like a serum rather than as an oil.

It is necessary to group the carrier oils or butters according to skin type first so you can limit your choices accordingly. After this, you can further limit your choice according to your further concerns.

Let us now discuss which oils are best for each specific concern.

For dry skin:

Fine lines and wrinkles

While all the oils listed above can be good for this problem because they are all very moisturizing, moisturizing the skin per se can be considered only a temporary solution to the signs of aging. What happens is the skin is temporarily plumped up so the fine lines and wrinkles become less obvious. However, if you really wish to diminish their appearance, here are your options starting from the best:

Rose hip oil – this oil contains vitamin C and A which are great antioxidants for the skin. Vitamin A encourages the skin to produce more collagen deep in the dermis resulting in smoother skin. It also gently exfoliates the skin resulting in a more radiant complexion. Vitamin C can also minimize dark spots.

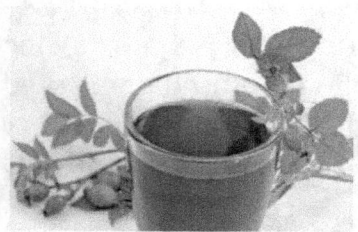

Argan oil – this oil is very high in vitamin E which is an excellent antioxidant for turning back the clock.

Avocado – this oil contains anti-inflammatory compounds called sterolins which help heal sun damage and age spots. If you are relatively young but see signs of skin damage, this might be a good choice for you to minimize premature aging.

Olive or coconut (your choice depending on your scent preference) – these oils are very emollient, but they have less anti-aging compounds compared to the above oils.

What about shea and cocoa butters? These are very good for moisturizing dry skin, but they are primarily used to make your natural skin care products more like a cream than a liquid oil. You must add other ingredients for additional benefits.

Dark spots

Rose hip oil is the best choice. (See above for the explanation.) Avocado oil can work for younger skins.

Fungal infections and dandruff

Coconut oil is best since it has natural anti-fungal properties. In fact, if you have used up your tea tree or lavender oil, you can just use coconut oil for fungal infections. It will take longer to heal without the essential oil, but all the same this proves how effective coconut oil is.

Eczema and psoriasis

As we have discussed, essential oils and carrier oils can only alleviate symptoms, not completely cure these ailments. Either olive or coconut oils are good choices to minimize the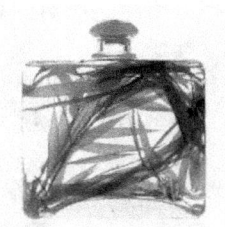

dryness of eczema and psoriasis.

Acne

If you have dry skin and acne, the best combination is coconut oil and tea tree, lavender or neem oil. Coconut oil has natural anti-bacterial properties which will keep inflammation at bay. You can alternate coconut oil with rose hip oil. The vitamin A in rose hip will help to exfoliate the skin of dead skin cells (one of the causes of acne) and will keep acne scars to a minimum.

For normal skin:

Fine lines and wrinkles

The oils fit for normal skin generally do not work well for minimizing fine lines and wrinkles, but they are good for preventing them.

Jojoba, sweet almond and apricot kernel oils can prevent fine lines and wrinkles only by moisturizing the skin. As discussed above, skin that is moisturized is well protected from the elements. These oils can replace sebum especially during the times when the skin produces less sebum like during the colder months.

You can also use these oils to lighten, i.e. make less emollient, the oils for dry skins to obtain their benefits.

What about beeswax? Beeswax is like cocoa or shea butter for dry skin. It is used to make a cream consistency, but it will not give you other benefits.

Dark spots

Castor oil can help heal dark spots given its healing abilities. However, it will work slower compared to rose hip oil. You can combine the two to lighten rose hip oil and to make your dark spots disappear faster.

Fungal infections and dandruff

Castor oil is the best choice for this problem because it contains the compound undecylenic acid which has anti-fungal properties.

Eczema and psoriasis

For alleviating dryness, jojoba, sweet almond or apricot kernel oil are good choices.

Acne

Castor oil contains anti-bacterial properties from ricinoleic acid. It will be less effective than coconut oil, but since it is lighter than the former, it can be a better choice for normal skin types.

For oily skin:

Oily skins can only use grape seed oil because using any other oil will result to excess greasiness. Fortunately, grape seed oil has a variety of benefits. It can help to regenerate the skin and minimize the signs of aging, alleviate the dryness of eczema and psoriasis and can help acne issues by making the oil glands produce less oil. However, it cannot help with fungal infections unless you use it with an essential oil like tea tree oil or lavender.

For hair issues:

Dry hair

Use the carrier oils prescribed for dry skin. However, avoid using the butters since they can leave a waxy film on the hair which can be difficult to remove.

Hair growth

Use castor oil as your carrier oil since this is proven to encourage hair to grow longer. You can also use pure castor oil to encourage eye lashes to grow longer. How long your lashes will grow still depends on your genetic make-up. Those who have naturally long lashes will still end up with longer lashes than those who have naturally short ones, but the point here is you will see an improvement. Also, you can use castor oil to encourage your brows to grow. This is particularly helpful if you accidentally shaved or plucked too much.

If you wish to try using castor oil on brows or lashes, Use a cotton bud to apply the castor oil and do not double dip into the bottle to avoid the spread of bacteria. Some people use their clean fingertip, but it is still more hygienic to use a clean cotton bud. Double dipping or using dirty tools can lead to eye infection especially for the lashes. You have to apply the castor oil on the eyelash roots, not on the eye lashes themselves. Do this carefully to avoid poking your eye, but don't be afraid if you get some oil on your eye. This will not be painful or hurt you in the long run; however, if you use contact lenses, remove them first before applying the oil. Also, don't re-insert your contact lenses. It is better to do this at night before sleeping so you don't have to use contact lenses anymore. To remove excess oil, pat tissue over your closed eye. You can expect to see results in 4 to 8 weeks assuming you do this at least once every day. To speed up things, you can apply castor oil at least 3 times throughout the day.

Do not add essential oil to the castor oil if you wish to use it on your lashes. Doing this can lead to irritation since it is an area which is very near the eye ball. You can use essential oil for the eye brows but just make sure that none gets into the eye. Sensitive eyes or eyes which easily tear up must avoid the essential oil especially lavender whose irritating fumes can reach the eye from the brows.

Castor oil was recommended for minimizing the signs of skin aging, but if it can also be used to encourage hair growth, will you end up with a beard? It sounds funny, but you don't have to worry about this. Castor oil only encourages hair growth but it does not create new hair follicles in the skin. It is true that a woman's facial skin is covered with tiny hairs, but these hair follicles can only grow short, tiny hairs. Even if castor oil encourages them to grow, they will only grow exactly what they are already growing: short, tiny, almost invisible hairs. It would be a different situation for a man whose facial hair follicles grow thick hair much like the head. Castor oil can help him to grow a longer beard should he wish to do so.

Lice

Removing lice will be easier if you use coconut oil as your carrier oil. It will drown the lice and dissolve the glue which adheres nits to the hair shaft.

Scalp psoriasis and dandruff

For scalp psoriasis, you can use any carrier oil which will help to dissolve the scales and alleviate dry, itchy skin.

As already mentioned above, coconut oil is good for dandruff which is caused by excess fungi on the scalp.

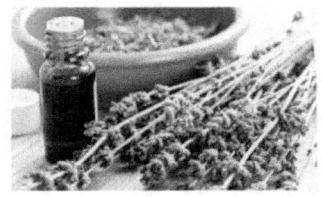

Chapter 5– Stress and Pain Relief

Another use for essential oils is to relieve stress and some minor aches and pains. For stress relief, usually essential oils are inhaled through oil burners or diffusers, dry evaporation, room sprays or steam inhalation. Oil burners are ceramic containers with a shallow bowl on top and space for a tea light underneath. The essential oil is placed on the shallow bowl, an equal amount of water is added and the tea light warms the solution to diffuse the scent. Essential oils should never be directly heated because this will change their scent. There are also electric appliances called diffusers which work on the same principle of warming the essential oil to release its scent. Alternatively, scented candles can be used.

For safety reasons, never leave an oil burner, diffuser or candle alone for several hours to avoid overheating. This can also change the scent of your essential oil.

For dry evaporation, the essential oil is applied to cotton, tissues or potpourri and the scent is allowed to disperse. This method will give a more subtle scent. You can also scent handkerchiefs and pillow cases. Room sprays work like body perfume. The essential oils are mixed with alcohol or water then this solution is sprayed to scent the room.

Lastly, steam inhalation works by inhaling the steam from hot water mixed with a few drops of essential oil like the steam facial described above. The last method is very potent because the nose is directly over the hot water. Only 1 to 2 drops of essential oils must be used or else the scent can be too overwhelming.

The method you choose will depend on your personal preferences. For example, while steam inhalation is the most potent, this can be too tedious for some. Busy people might find that room sprays or dry evaporation are more convenient.

As for the essential oil to choose, here are some options depending on your specific concern:

Anxiety – lavender, geranium, orange, patchouli

Depression – chamomile, jasmine, bergamot, rose

Insomnia – lavender, chamomile

To increase energy or to stimulate the mind – peppermint, rosemary, lemon, vanilla, grapefruit

An even more convenient way to decrease stress is to use essential oils as a perfume. If you are going to do this, make sure that you use true essential oils and not fragrance oils since you will apply this directly to your skin. Also, with the former the scent will be superior in quality.

You need to use carrier oils since directly applying essential oil to your skin will result in a too strong scent. Use half an ounce of neutral smelling vegetable oil like grape seed or sunflower oil then add the recommended amount of essential oils.

Here are some recipes for your stress-busting perfume:

Feminine	• 2 drops vanilla and 3 drops lavender
Citrus	• Equal amounts of lemon, grapefruit, and orange
Spicy	• 5 drops patchouli, 1 drop cinnamon

These are only recommended recipes but feel free to experiment to get your desired scent. When it comes to perfume, though the above are supposed to be for reducing stress, you still want to smell good. Allow the scent to combine with your own natural scent to see if it results in a pleasant fragrance. You might need to ask someone else to judge the resulting combination. It might take some time before you find the best recipe for yourself, but the above recipes are good starting points. The above combinations can also be used for your oil burner or room spray.

If you are going to use essential oils for pain relief like headaches and muscle pains, direct application to the painful area will be more effective. Peppermint, lavender and rosemary are the best choices for headaches. You can use the pure essential oil or combine it with carrier oil if you find the scent to be too strong. Apply a drop of this on the area of your head which feels painful. Take note that if you need to apply the essential oil on your temple or forehead, you might irritate your eyes. If so, you need to use a drop of carrier oil. Alternatively, you might wish to close your eyes and lie back for a while to hasten your healing.

For muscle aches, essential oils help to increase circulation and warm the muscle to sooth it. The best essential oils for general muscle pains include the following: basil, rosemary, clary sage, chamomile, lavender and elemi.

Sometimes, your muscle pains may be accompanied by inflammation. Examples of this situation include muscle strains or sprains. For these cases, essential oils which help reduce inflammation are better choices. These include: peppermint, lavender, clove, thyme and marjoram.

Lastly, essential oils can also help relax the muscles after a long day at work. The best way to relax the muscle is through massage. Combine 5 to 10 drops of the following essential oils with 1 cup of unscented massage oil: rosemary, peppermint, ginger, eucalyptus.

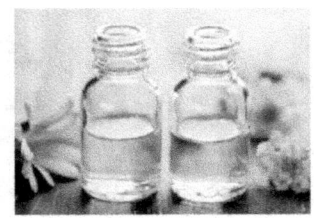

Chapter 6 – Weight Loss

Through aromatherapy, essential oils can also help boost your mood while you are trying to lose weight. Take note that the weight loss effect here is only indirect, more like a motivational speech than something which will actually make you burn excess calories. You cannot realistically expect essential oils to replace exercise and a healthy diet.

When using essential oils for weight loss, you can internally ingest 1 to 2 drops combined with a glass of water, tea or other liquid throughout the day or you can also sniff the scent. Do both these methods for the best results.

To be on the safe side, start with 1 drop and see if you experience any uncomfortable sensations or digestive problems. If 1 week has passed and you do not experience anything bad, move on to 2 drops. However, if you suddenly experience something bad, move back to 1 drop and stick with that amount.

Regarding the ingestion of essential oils, make sure that you are using true essential oils and not fragrance oils. The latter might be poisonous. Also, not all essential oils can be ingested. For example, tea tree oil is particularly dangerous and even a small amount can prove fatal if taken internally.

Make sure you are ingesting high quality essential oils which do not contain any impurities. The label should say 100% essential oil, and it should say that it has been tested for purity. This is an important precaution because impure essential oils can contain poisonous substances. This is also why you must start with using just 1 drop when trying this. If you wish to be even more cautious, ingest the drop of essential oil only every other day so you can observe the effect on your body. However, all the same, it is still best to ensure that the brand of essential oil you choose is pure and safe.

Those which are safe to ingest for weight loss include the following: grapefruit, lemon, peppermint and ginger. Take note that these essential oils are commonly used for cooking. To further ensure that you are ingesting safe essential oils, buy them from cooking supply stores rather than from your general essential oil store.

For variety, you can choose to cook with these essential oils (after you have checked for their safety). Add them to salad dressings, marinades or baked goods. Use a proportion which will ensure that the finished dish provides only 1 or 2 drops of essential oil per serving. For example, if the recipe provides 5 servings, add at most only 10 drops of essential oil.

Here are some further ideas:

- Add your choice of essential oil to your cake or muffin recipes. However, make sure that you avoid frosting the cake with high calorie frosting or whipped cream since you don't want to cancel out your weight loss efforts. You can also use no-calorie sweetener instead of sugar to further lessen the calories.

- Add a few drops of grapefruit or lemon essential oil to sauces to be served with fish.

- Mix 5 drops of lemon essential oil with 100 ml soy sauce. This will give the soy sauce a lemony aroma. It can be used as a dip for fish, sushi and for other uses where soy sauce is called for.

- Instead of lemon juice, use lemon essential oil. Use 4 drops to replace the juice from a medium lemon. Do the same for recipes calling for grapefruit juice, but use 6 drops since grapefruits are bigger. Make up for the lesser liquid by adding water. For ginger, use 1 drop for every inch square of ginger called for.

- Add a few drops of peppermint essential oil to your marinade for lamb. Lamb and mint are a classic combination.

- Add 3 drops of peppermint essential oil to non-fat whipped topping. This can be used as a minty topping for sugar-free hot chocolate or coffee. Alternatively, you can add 1 drop of peppermint to hot chocolate or coffee. This is a great drink for the winter holidays. Just ensure that you use no-calorie sweetener.

- Add 1 drop of peppermint essential oil to a cup of fruit salad for a refreshing zing which is especially good during the summer months. Don't add any sweetener.

- Add peppermint or ginger essential oil to lemonade or other summer drinks.

- Add ginger essential oil and ginger bread spices like cinnamon and nutmeg to your pancake or other quick bread recipes to give it a gingerbread twist.

- Add your choice of essential oil to sugar-free gelatin for a quick snack that helps with your weight loss.

- Use a few drops of your choice of essential oil to flavor merengue. A 1-inch merengue cookie, even if sugar is used, only provides 15 calories making it a great choice for times when you get a sugar craving.

Here are ideas for sniffing these essential oils to aid weight loss:

- Use an oil burner, diffuser or candle while exercising and during meals. Using room sprays require you to keep spraying while potpourri might not give a strong enough scent for your purposes.

- Sniff your choice of essential oil before every meal to help you control your appetite.

- Once you finish your food, sniff the essential oil again to avoid going back for seconds.

- If you are plagued by emotional eating, e.g. eating when stressed even if you are not hungry, sniff your essential oil.

Regularly ingesting these essential oils or regularly sniffing them can help to suppress your appetite and keep your metabolism under control. Again, take note that the operative word here is 'help.' You still have to continue with your usual reduced calorie diet and regular exercise regime.

Chapter 7 – Caution When Using Essential Oils

In this chapter, we will discuss some precautions you need to take when using essential oils. In the previous chapter, I assumed that you do not suffer from any health condition or are not pregnant. Also, I assume that you are an adult. Otherwise, there are certain precautions.

First, you need to make sure that you are not allergic to the essential oil or the carrier oils or butters you choose to use. Generally speaking, if you have a food allergy to a substance, you will also have a topical allergy to it. For example, if you are allergic to nuts, you will probably also get an allergic reaction when you apply shea butter (which comes from a nut) on your skin. There are cases where having a food allergy does not mean having a skin allergy, but you should be better safe than sorry. After all, you have a variety of other options besides shea butter.

Still regarding allergies, most people who do not have a lot of allergies will probably not be allergic to any of the essential oils listed in this book. However, if you have a lot of allergies, food or skin, then it is best to do a skin test before using an essential oil or a carrier oil or butter.

To do a skin test, get a small amount of the ingredients you wish to use. Apply a small amount on a hidden part of your body like the inside of the elbow, under the knee or behind the ear. Leave the substance for at least 24 hours. If irritation occurs, wash off the substance and apply some medicated cream which will help with the irritation. You must not use that substance in the future. Make sure that you test each substance individually otherwise you will not be able to know which caused the allergy, the essential oil or carrier oil.

Second, essential oils must be stored away from children and pets. They can be curious about these oils and inadvertently cause harm to themselves or others. Take note too that essential oils are flammable. If you are using them for aromatherapy, make sure that your oil burner or diffuser is safe. Low quality oil burners can allow the essential oil and water mixture to seep through the ceramic bowl and drip on the candle thus causing the flame to become bigger. If your oil burner is placed near curtains or furniture, it can result to a bigger fire.

Third, if you encounter an unfamiliar essential oil, do your research first to make sure you will not hurt yourself. It is best to stick to the tried and tested oils. Why should you try out an unfamiliar essential oil if you know that what you are currently using is working? Some can also be toxic like wormwood which can result in hallucinations and pennyroyal which can cause miscarriage, organ damage and even death. These names are usually unfamiliar to many people, but just in case you encounter them in the store, make sure you avoid them. Reputable stores will likely not sell these to people, but some stores might carry them for experienced users of these essential oils.

Fourth, always start with the smallest recommended dose when trying out an essential oil even if they are already familiar like lavender. This is just to avoid unforeseen complications. Once you are sure that you will experience no irritation or discomfort, you can progress to the higher amounts.

Fifth, it is best to avoid using essential oils for newborns and very young infants. They still have very sensitive skins which may be irritated if applied with essential oils. If you need something for certain problems like eczema, it is better to use coconut oil which is proven to be gentle enough for baby's skin. Apricot kernel oil is also a good choice for young skin. At any rate, very young children are usually still not plagued by the issues discussed here.

Sixth, do not assume that all essential oils can be used for aromatherapy. Some essential oils like neem smell bad and may make you nauseous.

Seventh, pregnant and nursing women must be careful when using essential oils. Many are not safe for them even if they are used for skin conditions or fragrance because they can be absorbed by the skin and brought into the bloodstream or milk glands where they will eventually affect the fetus or infant. Here are the essential oils which pregnant women can safely use: rose, chamomile, jasmine, lavender, geranium, sandalwood, frankincense. Generally speaking, pregnant women should not ingest essential oils for whatever reason until they have given birth.

You might ask: even perfume is not allowed? Cologne or eau de toilette which contains only a very small percentage of essential oil compared to alcohol is safe. What I am referring to above is the pure essential oil. You can try using it with diluted with carrier oil, but why would you risk your health and your baby's?

Eighth, those who suffer from certain medical conditions **should avoid** certain essential oils used in any way, including aromatherapy:

Epilepsy – rosemary, sage, camphor and fennel (These can encourage seizures.)

High blood pressure – rosemary, sage, thyme

Asthma – marjoram

Hepatitis or cirrhosis – avoid **all** essential oils

Ninth, certain essential oils must not be used in the *long term* or else they can be toxic due to a build-up of harmful toxins in the body. These include cinnamon, juniper, coriander, eucalyptus, turmeric and laurel.

Tenth, if you will be exposed to the sun, avoid using these oils since they can cause dark spots to form: bergamot, cedar wood, ginger, grapefruit, and patchouli. If you use any of these for skin care or other purposes, use them at night or else on an area that is not touched by sun light.

Eleventh, take note of the scent and appearance of the essential oil when fresh. If they change scent, color and viscosity, toss them. Citrus essential oils usually last for only a year while flowers last for up to 5 years if they are stored properly. Those with the heavier scents like sandalwood, patchouli and frankincense can last up to several years.

This is the reason why essential oils are usually sold in small bottles. Since they are concentrated, you only need to use a small amount. Keeping a large bottle, unless you have many uses for it, will only result in waste.

Twelfth, if you are in doubt, don't. If you need to do more research, do so. It is important to understand that essential oils are medicines. Even if they are not regulated in the same way as prescription medication, they can still cause harm if misused. If you need further advice on how to use certain essential oils, go beyond books and internet sources by consulting an actual expert. Just like how you need to go to an actual doctor if your sickness is serious instead of just depending on books or internet sources, a direct discussion with an essential oil expert will allow you to voice out all your concerns. It will also allow the expert to judge which essential oil is best for your specific situation after considering all relevant information like allergies, past and present medical conditions and personal preferences.

Conclusion

Thank you again for downloading this book!

I hope this book was able to help you to use essential oils for your various ailments.

The next step is to try out the tips for yourself and experiment to know what works for you. As long as you are careful and always test your new concoctions, you can be sure that essential oils will only give you many benefits.

Finally, if you enjoyed this book, please take the time to share your thoughts and post a review on Amazon. We do our best to reach out to readers and provide the best value we can. Your positive review will help us achieve that. It'd be greatly appreciated!

Thank you and good luck!

Check Out My Other Books

Below you'll find some of my other popular books that are popular on Amazon and Kindle as well. Simply click on the links below to check them out. Alternatively, you can visit my author page on Amazon to see other work done by me.

Coconut Oil for Easy Weight Loss: A Step by Step Guide for Using Virgin Coconut Oil for Quick and Easy Weight Loss

http://www.amazon.com/Coconut-Oil-Easy-Weight-Loss-ebook/dp/B00JG8H8DE

Superfoods that Kickstart Your Weight Loss Learn How to Use 30 Superfoods to Boost Weight Loss, Immunity and to Live a Healthier Lifestyle

http://www.amazon.com/Superfoods-Kickstart-Healthier-Lifestyle-Healthstyle-ebook/dp/B00JNAPM9M

Carrier Oils for Beginners: Discover the Characteristics and Beauty and Health Benefits of Carrier Oils For mixing Aromatherapy Essential Oils

http://www.amazon.com/Carrier-Oils-Beginners-Characteristics-Aromatherapy-ebook/dp/B00K88GI2S

Natural Homemade Cleaning Recipes For Beginners: Essential Oil Recipes For Household Cleaning, Laundry & Toxic Free Living

http://www.amazon.com/Natural-Homemade-Cleaning-Recipes-Beginners-ebook/dp/B00K87UBQI

The Best Secrets of Natural Remedies: The Ultimate Guide to Natural Remedies to Prevent and Cure Illnesses, Cold and Flu for Your Family

http://www.amazon.com/Best-Secrets-Natural-Remedies-Illnesses-ebook/dp/B00JNDCOCM

The Hypothyroidism Handbook: An Everyday Guide to Natural Solutions of living with Hypothyroidism including increased energy, lasting weight loss, and general well-being

http://www.amazon.com/Hypothyroidism-Handbook-Solutions-including-increased-ebook/dp/B00JNIGIV0

The Hyperthyroidism Handbook: An Everyday Guide to Natural Solutions of Living with Hyperthyroidism including Weight Gain, Increased Energy and General Well-being

http://www.amazon.com/Hyperthyroidism-Handbook-Solutions-including-Hypothyroidism-ebook/dp/B00JOHU5SM

Essential Oils & Weight Loss for Beginners: Ultimate Guide to Losing Weight, Increasing Energy, Balancing Metabolism & Appetite Using Essential Oils & Aromatherapy

http://www.amazon.com/Essential-Oils-Weight-Loss-Beginners-ebook/dp/B00JOFOWP6

Top Essential Oil Recipes: A Recipe Guide Of Natural, Non-Toxic Aromatherapy & Essential Oils for Healing Common Ailments, Beauty, Stress & Anxiety

http://www.amazon.com/Top-Essential-Oil-Recipes-Aromatherapy-ebook/dp/B00JY434E2

Soap Making For Beginners: A Guide to Making Natural Homemade Soaps from Scratch, Includes Recipes and Step by Step Processes for Making Soaps

http://www.amazon.com/Soap-Making-Beginners-Homemade-Processes-ebook/dp/B00JYKH75I

Body Butters For Beginners: Proven Secrets To Making All Natural Body Butters For Rejuvenating And Hydrating Your Skin

http://www.amazon.com/Body-Butters-Beginners-Rejuvenating-Hydrating-ebook/dp/B00K6LVV6A

Apple Cider Vinegar For Beginners: Proven Secrets Using Apple Cider Vinegar For Health, Weight Loss, and Skin Care

http://www.amazon.com/Apple-Cider-Vinegar-Beginners-Aromatherapy-ebook/dp/B00K6YY6HI

Homemade Body Scrubs & Masks For Beginners: 50 Proven All Natural, Easy Recipes For Body & Facial Masks To Exfoliate Nourish, & Care For Your Skin

http://www.amazon.com/Homemade-Body-Scrubs-Masks-Beginners-ebook/dp/B00K79D4SY

Box Set #2: Essential Oils & Weight Loss For Beginners (Ultimate Guide to Losing Weight, Increasing Energy, Balancing Metabolism & Appetite Using Essential Oils & Aromatherapy) + Top Essential Oil Recipes (A Recipe Guide of Natural, Non-Toxic Aromatherapy & Essential Oils for Healing Common Ailments, Beauty, Stress & Anxiety)

http://www.amazon.com/ESSENTIAL-OILS-BOX-SET-Aromatherapy-ebook/dp/B00K7Q8HRK

Box Set#3: Coconut Oil for Easy Weight Loss(A Step by Step Guide for Using Virgin Coconut Oil for Quick and Easy Weight Loss) + Apple Cider Vinegar(Proven Secrets Using Apple Cider Vinegar for Health, Weight Loss, and Skin Care)

http://www.amazon.com/Box-Set-Beginners-Aromatherapy-Essential-ebook/dp/B00K9TEGUW

Box Set #4: Body butters For Beginners(Proven Secrets To Making All Natural Body Butters For Rejuvenating And Hydrating Your Skin) & Top Essential Oil Recipes: A Recipe Guide Of Natural, Non-Toxic Aromatherapy & Essential Oils for Healing Common Ailments, Beauty, Stress & Anxiety

http://www.amazon.com/Box-Set-Butters-Beginners-Essential-ebook/dp/B00KA02F4Y

Box Set #5: Soap Making For Beginners(A Guide to Making Natural Homemade Soaps from Scratch, Includes Recipes and Step by Step Processes for Making Soaps) + Homemade Body Scrubs & Masks For Beginners(50 Proven All Natural, Easy Recipes For Body Scrub & Facial Masks To Exfoliate, Nourish, & Care For Your Skin)

http://www.amazon.com/Box-Set-Beginners-Homemade-Recipes-ebook/dp/B00K9U3I2I

Box Set #6: Body Butters for Beginners (Proven Secrets To Making All Natural Body Butters For Rejuvenating And Hydrating Your Skin) +Homemade Body Scrubs & Masks For Beginners(50 Proven All Natural, Easy Recipes For Body Scrub & Facial Masks To Exfoliate, Nourish, & Care For Your Skin)

http://www.amazon.com/Box-Set-Beginners-Exfoliating-Moisturizing-ebook/dp/B00K9U3Y40

Box Set #7: Top Essential Oils (A Recipe Guide Of Natural, Non-Toxic Aromatherapy & Essential Oils For Healing, Common Ailments, Beauty, Stress & Anxiety) & The Best Secrets Of Natural Remedies (The Ultimate Guide to Natural Remedies to Prevent and Cure Illnesses, Cold and Flu for Your Family)

http://www.amazon.com/BOX-SET-Essential-Recipes-Remedies-ebook/dp/B00K9WPMQG

Box Set #8: Natural Homemade Cleaning Recipes For Beginners (Essential Oil Recipes for Household Cleaning, Laundry & Toxic Free Living) + Top Essential Oils (A Recipe Guide Of Natural, Non-Toxic Aromatherapy & Essential Oils For Healing, Common Ailments, Beauty, Stress & Anxiety)

http://www.amazon.com/BOX-SET-Beginners-Essential-Aromatherapy-ebook/dp/B00KAMNGBS

Box Set #9: Essential Oils & Weight Loss for Beginners (Ultimate Guide to Losing Weight, Increasing Energy, Balancing Metabolism & Appetite Using Essential Oils & Aromatherapy) + Carrier Oils for Beginners (Discover the Characteristics and Beauty and Health Benefits of Carrier Oils for Mixing Aromatherapy Essential Oils)

http://www.amazon.com/BOX-SET-Essential-Beginners-Aromatherapy-ebook/dp/B00KAODL6Q

Box Set #10: The Hyperthyroidism Handbook (An Everyday Guide to Natural Solutions of Living with Hyperthyroidism including Weight Gain, Increased Energy and General Well-being) + The Hyperthyroidism Handbook (Everyday Guide to Natural

Solutions of Living With Hypothyroidism Including Increased Energy, Lasting Weight Loss, and General Well-Being)

http://www.amazon.com/BOX-SET-10-Hyperthyroidism-Hypothyroidism-ebook/dp/B00KAKMSBY

Box Set #11: Carrier Oils For Beginners (Discover the Characteristics and Beauty and Health Benefits of Carrier Oils for Mixing Aromatherapy Essential Oils) + Essential Oils & Aromatherapy for Beginners (Secrets to Beauty, Health and Weight Loss Using Proven Essential Oil and Aromatherapy Recipes

http://www.amazon.com/BOX-SET-Beginners-Essential-Aromatherapy-ebook/dp/B00KAONEQ8

Box Set 12: Essential Oils & Weight Loss For Beginners: (Ultimate Guide to Losing Weight, Increasing Energy, Balancing Metabolism & Appetite Using Essential Oils & Aromatherapy) + Top Essential Oil Recipes (A Recipe Guide of Natural, Non-Toxic Aromatherapy & Essential Oils for Healing Common Ailments, Beauty, Stress & Anxiety) + Carrier Oils For Beginners (Discover the Characteristics & Beauty & Health Benefits of Carrier Oils for Mixing Aromatherapy Essential Oils) + Essential Oils & Aromatherapy For Beginners (Secrets to Beauty & weight Loss Using Proven Essential Oil & Aromatherapy Recipes) + Natural Homemade Cleaning Recipes For Beginners (Essential Oil Recipes for Household Cleaning, Laundry & Toxic Free Living)

http://www.amazon.com/BOX-SET-12-Essential-Aromatherapy-ebook/dp/B00KCBCHE4

Box Set #13: Superfoods That Kickstart Your Weight Loss (Learn How to Use 30 Superfoods to Boost Weight Loss, Immunity and to Live a Healthier Lifestyle) + Essential Oils & Aromatherapy For Beginners (Secrets to Beauty, Health and Weight Loss Using Proven Essential Oil and Aromatherapy Recipes) + Body Butters For Beginners (Proven Secrets To Making All Natural Body Butters For Rejuvenating And Hydrating Your Skin) + Soap Making For Beginners (A Guide to Making Natural Homemade Soaps from Scratch, Includes Recipes and Step by Step Processes for Making Soaps) + Homemade Body Scrubs For Beginners (50 Proven All Natural, Easy Recipes For Body Scrub & Facial Masks To Exfoliate, Nourish, & Care For Your Skin)

http://www.amazon.com/BOX-SET-Superfoods-Kickstart-Aromatherapy-ebook/dp/B00KC8G6DK/

Box Set 14: Essential Oils & Weight Loss for Beginners (Ultimate Guide to Losing Weight, Increasing Energy, Balancing Metabolism & Appetite Using Essential Oils & Aromatherapy) + Apple Cider Vinegar for Beginners (Proven Secrets Using Apple Cider Vinegar for Health, Weight Loss, and Skin Care) + Body Butters For Beginners (Proven Secrets To Making All Natural Body Butters For Rejuvenating And Hydrating Your Skin) + Homemade Body Scrubs & Masks for Beginners (50 Proven All Natural, Easy Recipes for Body Scrub & Facial Masks to Exfoliate, Nourish, & Care for Your Skin) + Coconut Oil for Easy Weight Loss (A Step by Step Guide for Using Virgin Coconut Oil for Quick and Easy Weight Loss)

http://www.amazon.com/BOX-SET-Essential-Beginners-Aromatherapy-ebook/dp/B00KEDO68U

If the links do not work, for whatever reason, you can simply search for these titles on the Amazon website to find them.